MIND *flip*

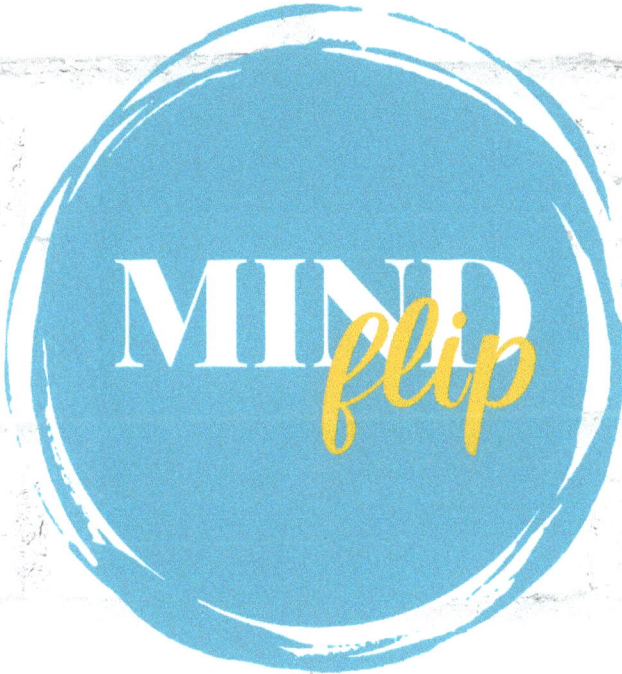

EMOTIONAL TOOLBOX AND POSITIVE
MINDSET FOR KIDS AND TEENS

Heidi Horne

Growing up and living in today's worries?

Here are ways to cope and build up your emotional tool-box.

Flip your mind with these easy and short exercises short (5-10minutes) and flip the negative into a positive mindset.

This book is aimed for 8-16 year olds, however it can be used for any age. Teach your mums, dads, caregivers, teachers and grandparents. I am pretty sure they could use some of these tips too!

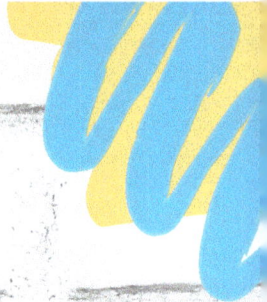

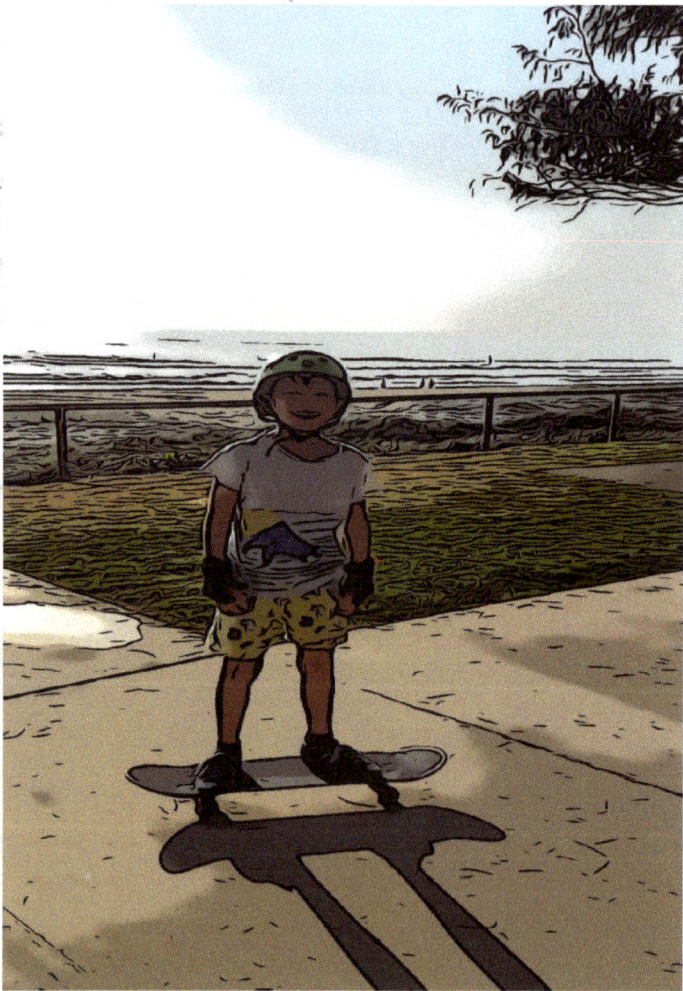

Introduce simple yoga, meditation and breathing techniques into your day.

Be your own best friend, not your worst enemy!

Create a daily healthy habit to check in on your mental health and use your emotional toolbox.
Small changes to make a big difference.
Introduce simple yoga, meditation and breathing techniques for any time and anyone.

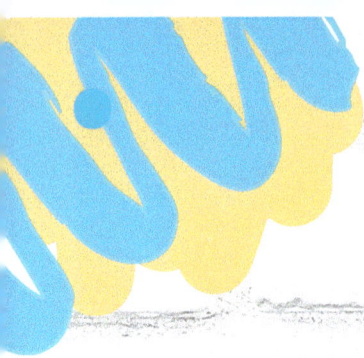

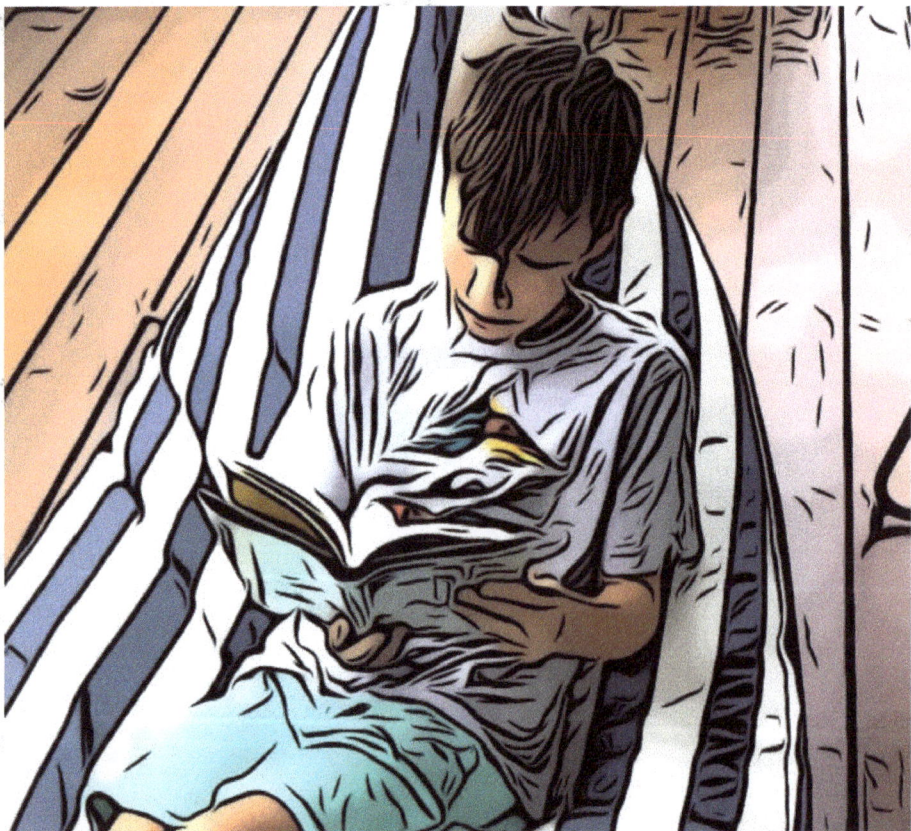

BENEFITS FROM THIS BOOK

- Create energy

- Feel connected and calm

- Be present

- Help release stress

- Tips for anxiety and fear

- Help with good nights sleep

- Introduce meditation and yoga

- Breathe more deeply

- Daily check in with self

FLIP TO THE PAGE NUMBER IF FEELING...

FEELING STRESSED?

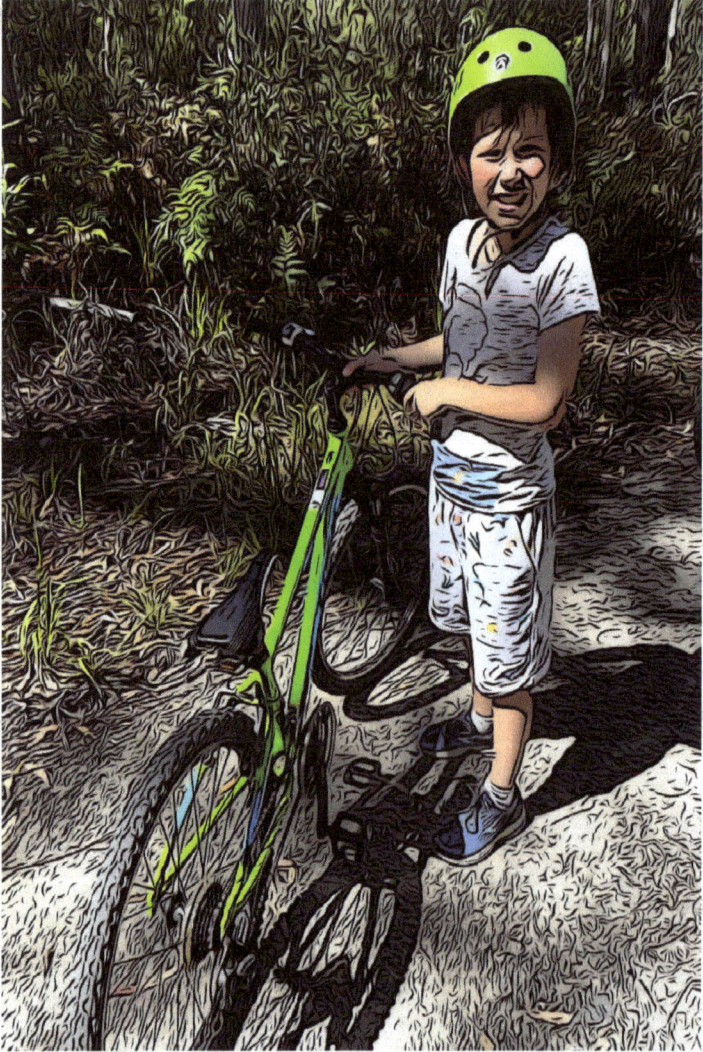

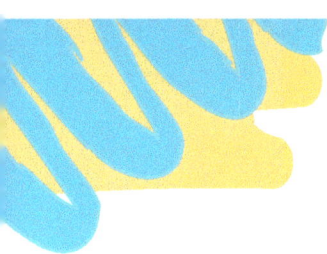

POSITIVE STRESS: helps motivates us, focuses our energy, feels exciting, allows us to rise to the challenge, improves our performance. It is usually fleeting and fine from time to time. A sign body performing at it's best.

When we feel stressed constantly, that is when problems arise.

NEGATIVE STRESS: feels unpleasant, takes us beyond our coping skills, inhibits our performance, and operates from fear and anxiety.

Stress makes us feel overwhelmed, negative thoughts and can also make us feel angry.

Some stress is good, it allows us to do well and keeps us performing at our best. Too much is not.

Can't stop stress in our life, however, we can change how we react to those situations.

EYE OF THE STORM MEDITATION

Make yourself comfortable. Sit cross-leg on the floor, or lie down flat on the back, with arms and legs not crossed.

Close your eyes have some slow deep breaths and once you feel calm we will use our imagination.

Imagine there is a hurricane storm.

You are in the eye of the storm, the quiet centre of the hurricane where it is peaceful.

You can see all the moving and changing around you but you are calm and in control where it is still and quiet.

This is like life. There will always be stresses and chaos happening around you, but you can choose not to get involved, and observe and be calm and peaceful in the middle.

MINI REWARD BREAKS

If studying for school, make sure you treat yourself with a mini reward at a set time
ie. every 20 minutes.

These can be things like going outside, hugging your pet, listening to your favourite song, or having a snack.

Avoid scrolling on the phone as the time will fly by and will be hard to get back to school-work.

LOW IN ENERGY?

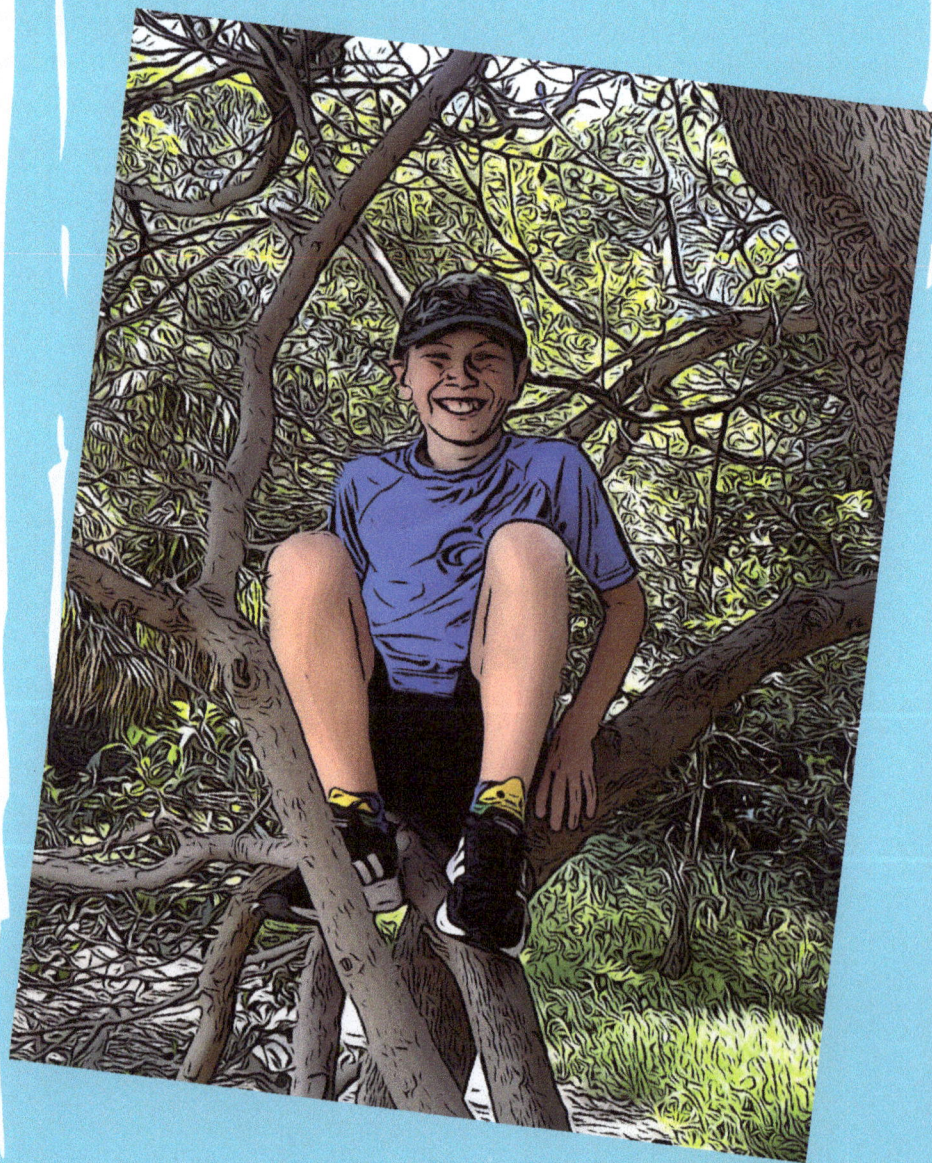

INCREASE YOUR ENERGY IN THE DAY

- Eat your fruits and vegetables
- Take some slow deep breaths
- Take a mini break and stretch
- Keep drinking that water
- Deep breaths
- Get upside down
- Sit outside if you can for lunch and recess and when you get home after school
- Spend time in nature and the fresh air

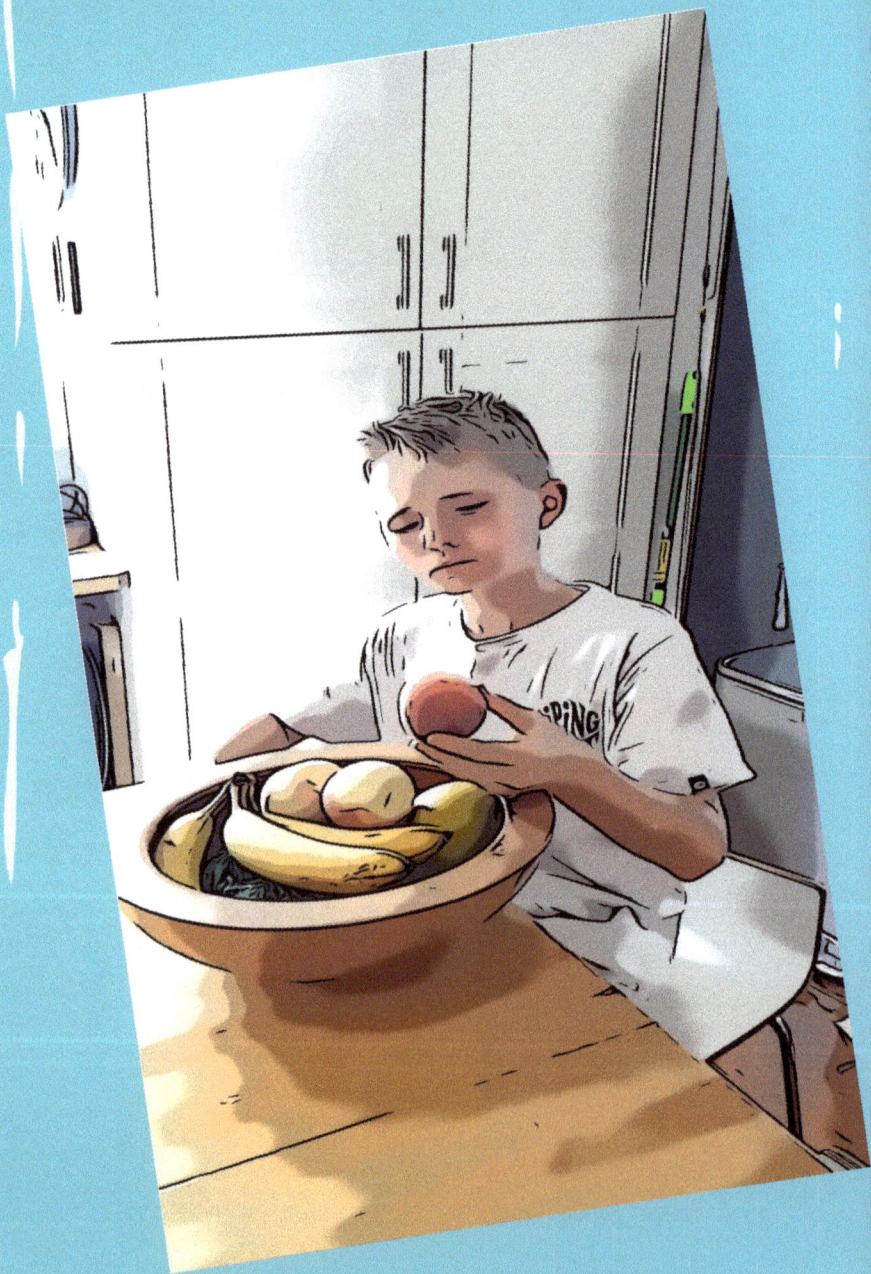

ENERGY FOODS

Add some of these natural energy boosters to your daily intake:

- Bananas
- Fatty fish – like salmon
- Brown rice
- Sweet potatoes
- Eggs
- Quinoa
- Green leafy vegetables
- Avocados
- Berries
- Nuts
- Green tea

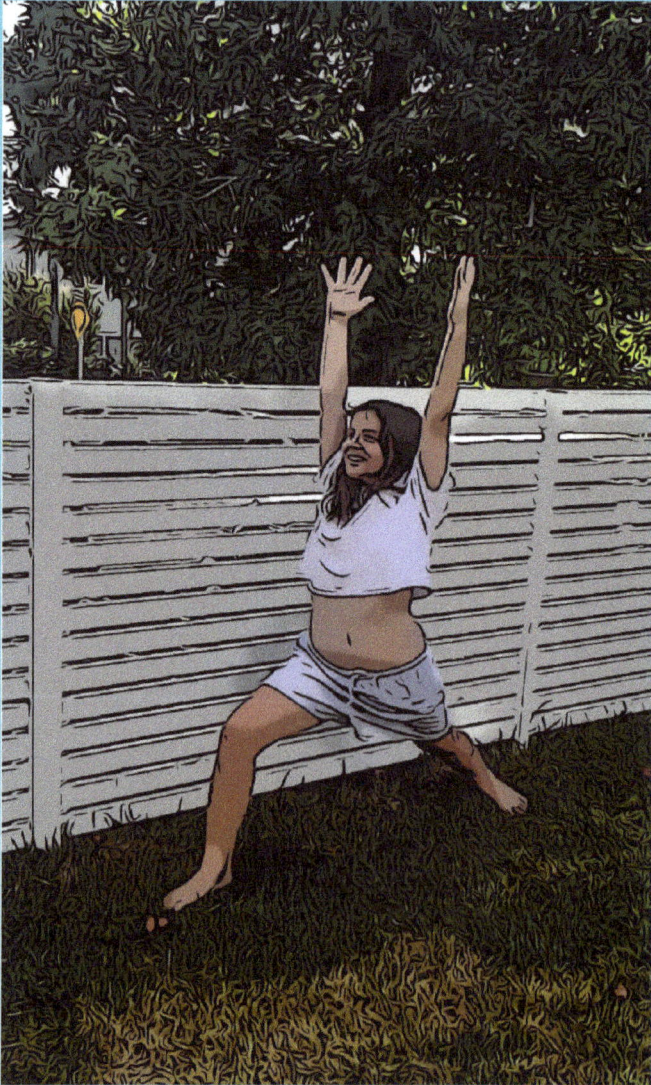

TRY THIS

DO SOME SUN SALUTES

Sometimes, the last thing you feel like doing is exercise when you are tired. However, you only need a few rounds of sun salutes (5-10 minutes) to get the benefits and give yourself a natural energy boost!

It gets the blood pumping and helps your circulation while stretching the whole body, which gives you amazing positive energy for your body and your mind. There have also been studies done to show that this yoga exercise can help with anxiety and depression, along with your memory – a great one before any exams!

Do a sun salute along with me. Use this link for short video to get you learning the basics: www.bit.ly/SUNSALUTES

FEELING NEGATIVE?

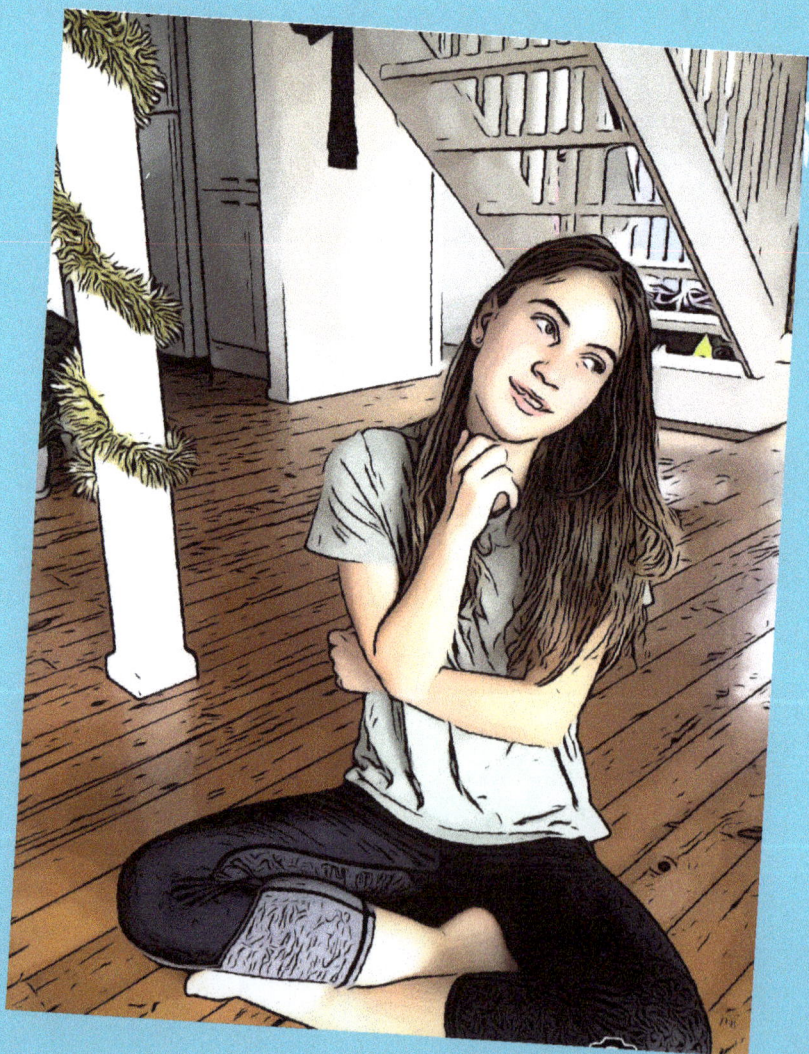

NEGATIVE MINDSET THOUGHTS

Do you have negative thoughts?

- Negative thoughts are when you have constant self critism

- More you hear them, the more you believe it

- They can make you feel low and depressed

- Can affect how you are with your friends and family

- When you are negative with yourself, you become needy, grumpy and negative with others

- How do you talk to yourself? Notice when you have negative thoughts and replace them with positive affirmations instead.

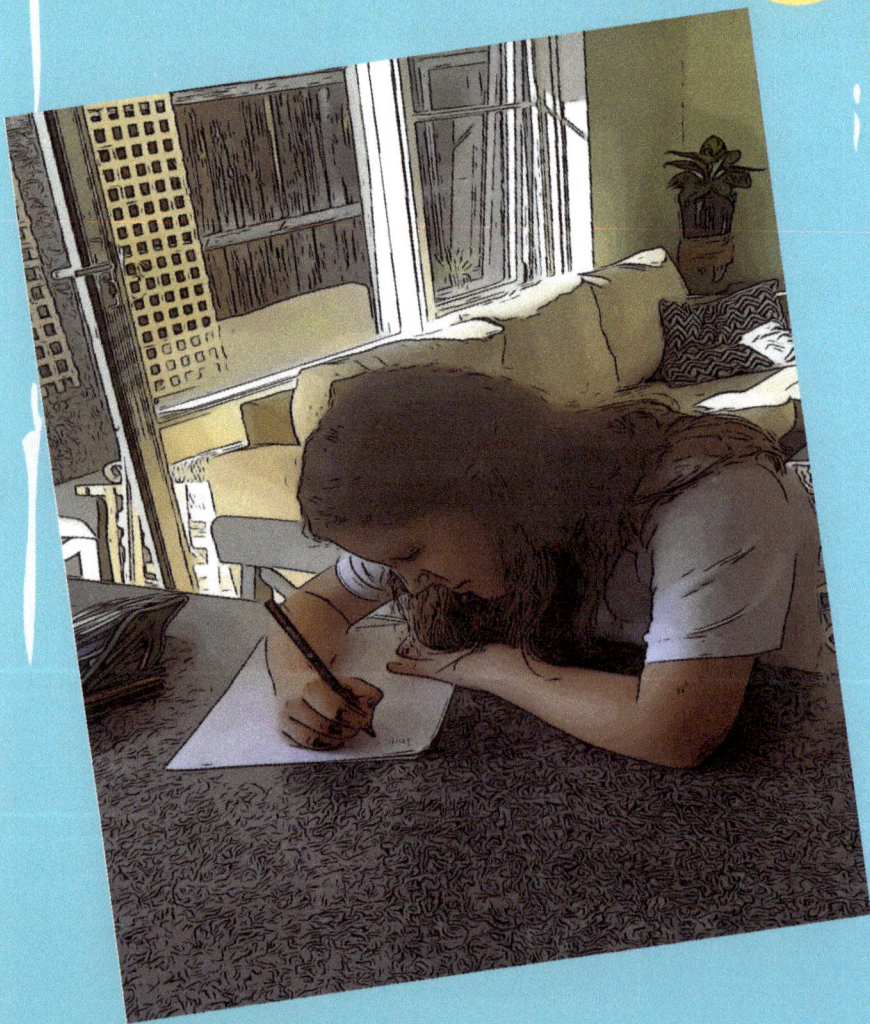

HERE ARE SOME EXAMPLES OF NEGATIVE SELF-TALK

Any of these sound familiar?

- I am no good at maths

- I will never be able to play tennis

- Everyone is better than me

- My brother is smarter than me, I am the dumb one in the family

- I will never remember enough

- I am ugly and never wear the right clothes

- I will never be picked for the Div 1 soccer team

- I am hopeless at drawing

- I will always be nervous and stuff up my public speaking

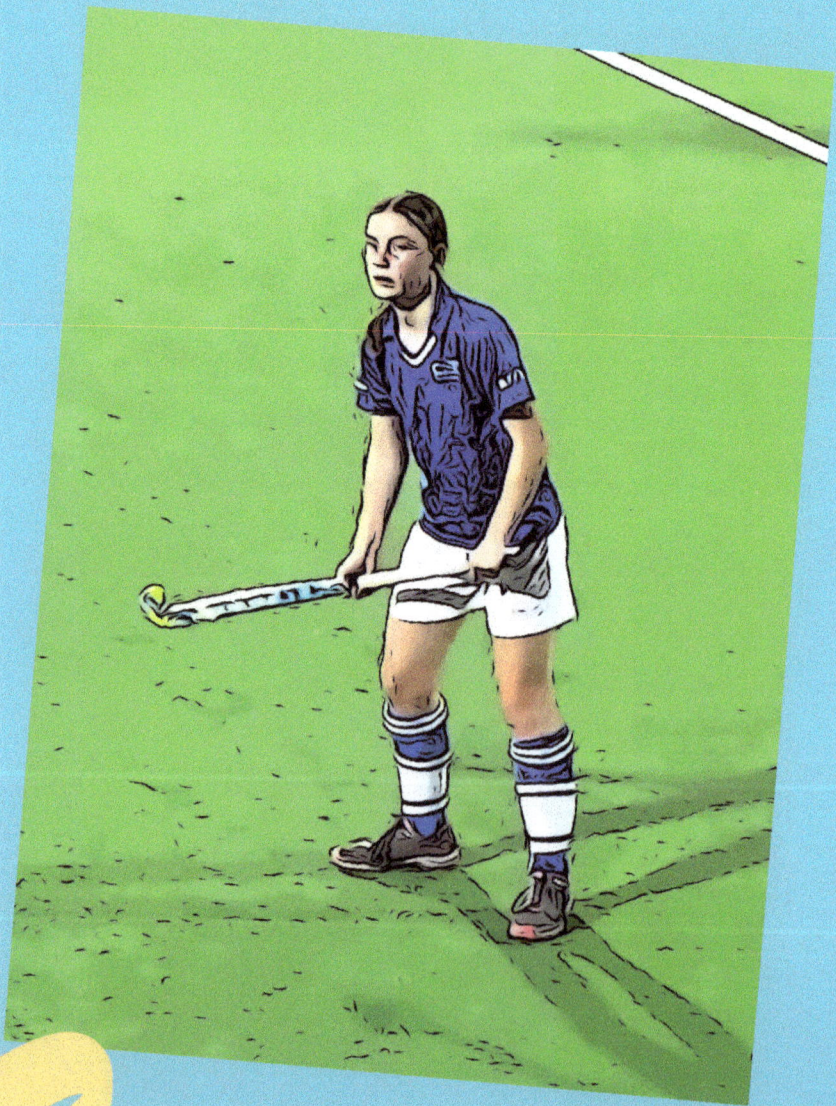

- Play the game – swap a negative for a positive.
- The next time you hear you speak to yourself in a negative way, swap it for a positive!
- Even if you do not believe it to be true right now.
- The more you say it, the more you will believe it. For example, you might say "I am no good at hockey"

  Instead say "I am a good hockey player"
- Say it until you believe it. If you can, say it out-loud and over and over!
- Make it a game, and do this each time you say something negative about yourself.

FEEL LIKE YOU ARE NOT GOOD ENOUGH?

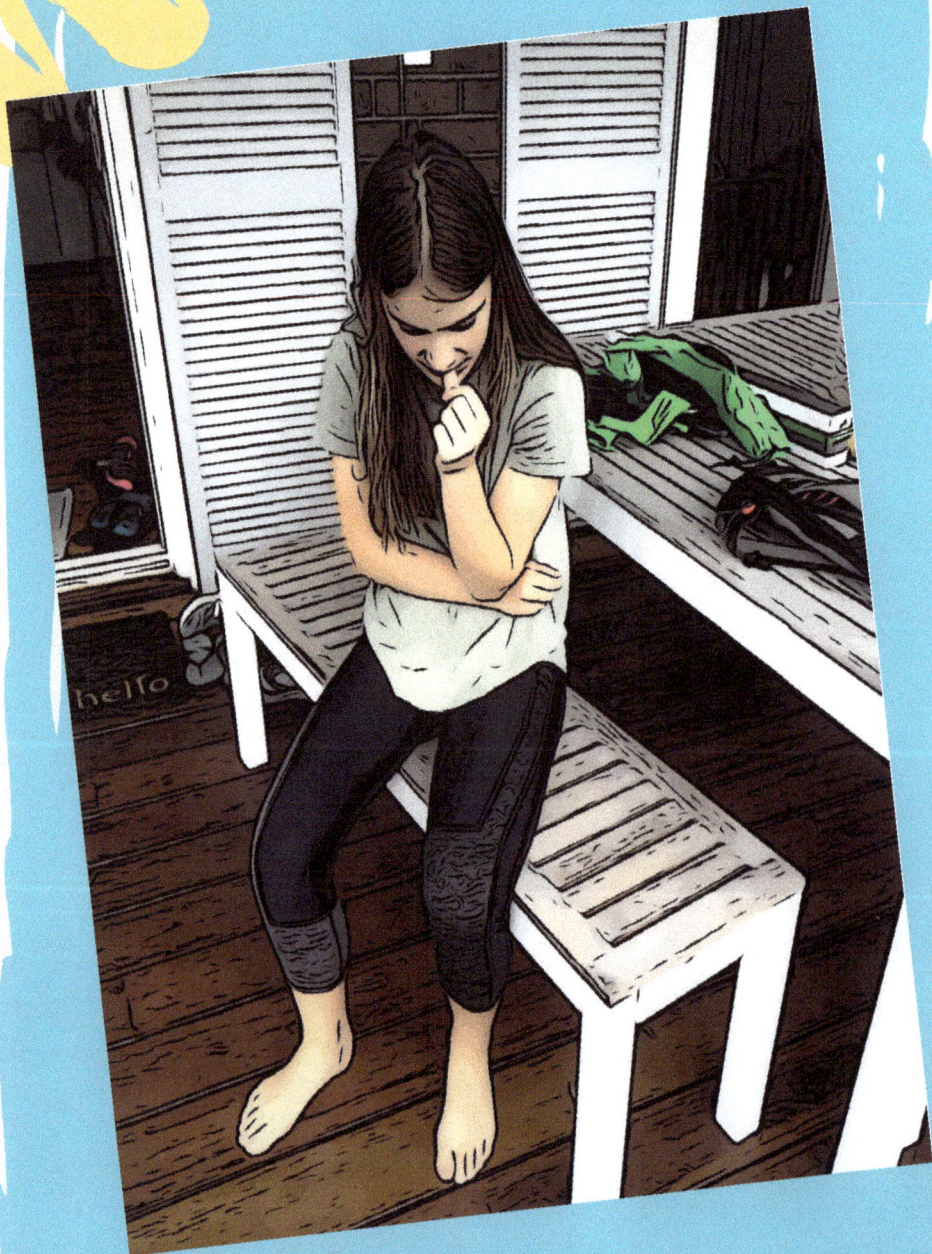

- Are you upset about the way you look? Feel you are not good enough?
- Take a moment to hear how you are talking to yourself.
- Negative thoughts are where you have Constant self-criticism.
- We talk to ourselves more than anyone else in the world – more than we talk to our parents or friends.
- Are you talking to yourself as a friend, and supporting yourself?
- The more you hear negative self-talk, the more you believe it.
- Can make you feel low and depressed.
- Can affect how you are with friends and family. When you are negative with yourself, you become needy and negative with others
- Take the time to listen. Be your own best friend, rather than the worst enemy.

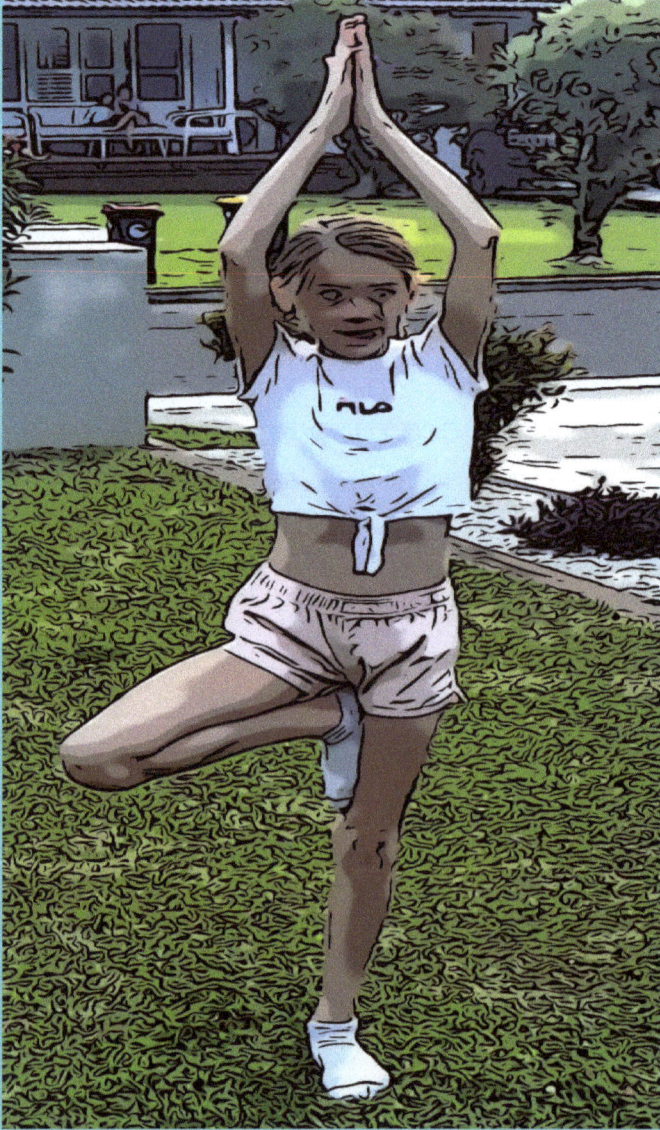

TRY A BALANCE

Try something challenging, such as a yoga balance.

Start with Tree Pose.

Balance on your right foot and bring your left foot up onto your ankle, calf or thigh. Arms out to the side or up in the air.

Notice how you talk to yourself in the pose.

Are you telling yourself off and saying 'I can't do this or 'I am no good. Instead, tell yourself how great you are (even if you fall out after a few seconds!)

POP IT ON A BUBBLE

During the day, when you notice you have a negative thought about yourself. Imagine you are picking up the thought and putting it in a bubble and float it out of your mind.

It may seem silly, but the more you do it, the less negative thoughts you will continue to have.

ANXIOUS ABOUT SCHOOL

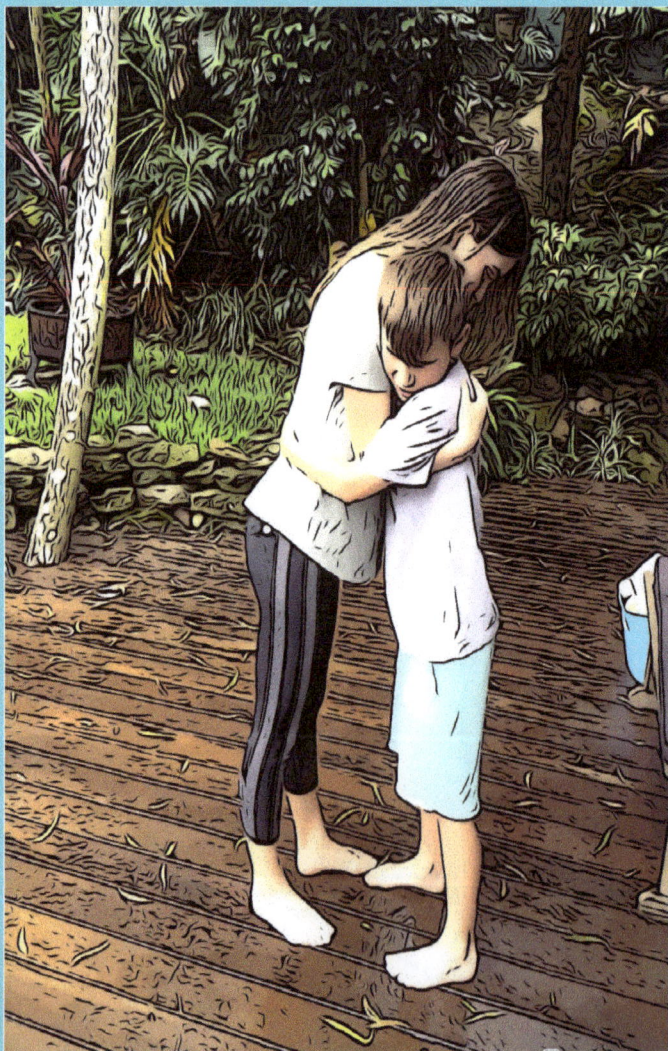

WHAT IS IT LIKE TO FEEL ANXIOUS

- Feels unpleasant
- It is thinking something bad is going to happen.
- You may feel tightness in the chest or pounding heart, or butterflies in the tummy.
- It is the habit of the mind to project a negative future for yourself.
- What makes it worse? Tiredness, Stress, Crowds / Loneliness

- Hug someone you love

- Spend time with a pet

- Listen to your favorite music

- Practice deep breathing exercises

- Reduce caffeine

- Do something for others – give back

- Exercise – yoga, go for a walk, or run

- Have a laugh

- Learn about your triggers

- Take time out for yourself – go to the park or read

- Set aside time to write worries down

- Listen to a guided meditation

BREATHING EXERCISES FOR ANXIETY

- Crocodile Breath: Lie face down with your feet wide and your forehead resting on your hands. Close your eyes and breath in and out slowly through the nostrils. Focus on your breathing and your belly going in and out onto the floor underneath you. Stay as long as you need to.

- Calming Words: Get comfortable sitting cross leg on the floor, or lying on back with arms and legs uncrossed. Focus on the breath in and out through the nostrils. Then add some words with the breath to make you feel calm.

- Some examples, as you INHALE (breath in) say I AM CALM, and as you EXHALE (breath out), say I AM IN CONTROL or even I AM RELAXED.

TROUBLE SLEEPING

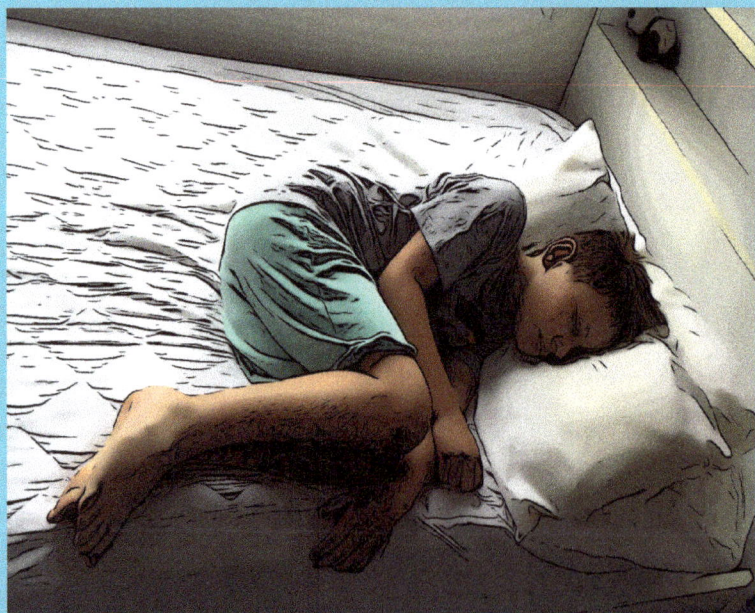

WHY IS SLEEP SO IMPORTANT?

- Operate at your best self

- Lack of sleep, basic tasks difficult

- Proper sleep contributes to wellness

- Body and brain have a chance to recover

- Balance out school/screen with rest and sleep and feel the difference

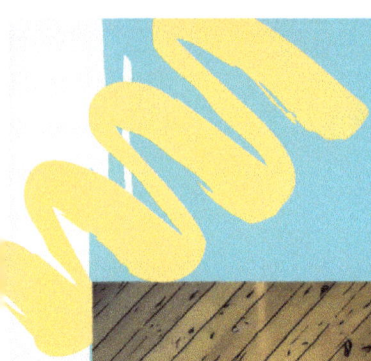
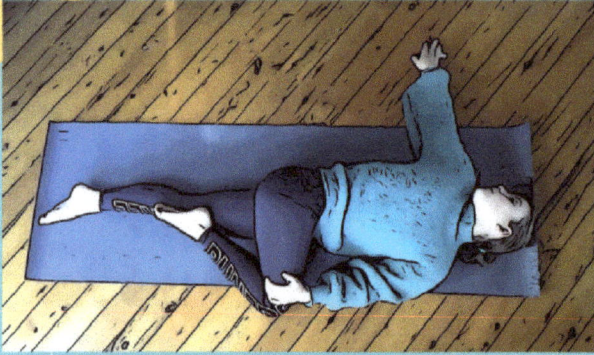
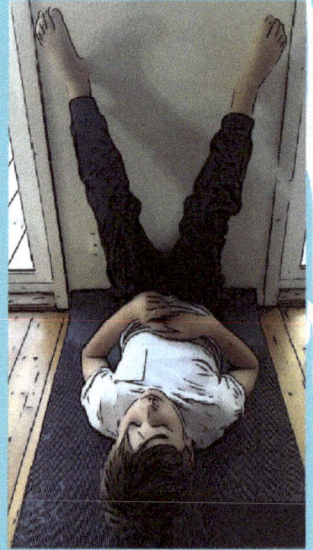
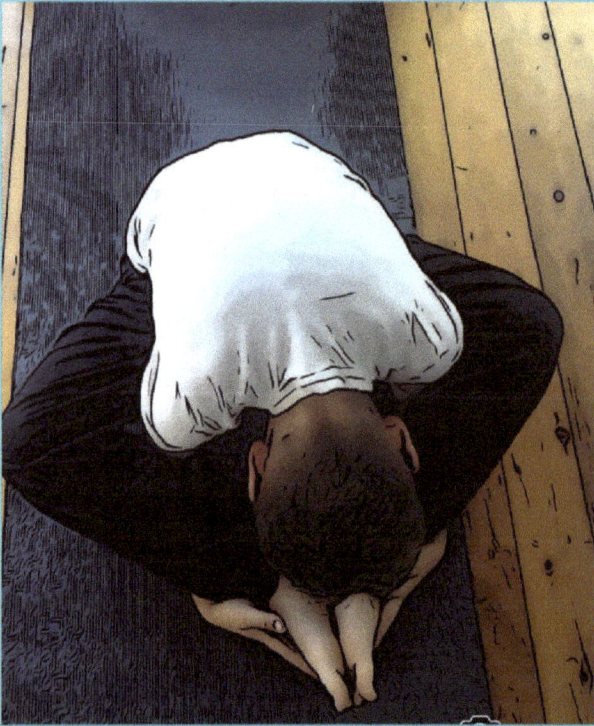
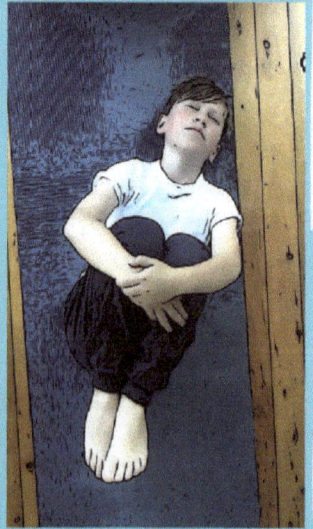

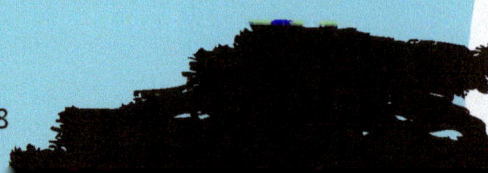

YOGA POSES TO HELP YOU SLEEP

- **Sleeping Turtle**
  Sitting down, bring soles of feet together with knees bent. Slide arms under ankles and hold outside of feet with hands. Slowly lower forehead to heels and hold for 5-10 breaths.

- **Knee to Chest**
  Lying on your back, hug the knees, and gently rock side to side, and release your back.

- **Reclining Twist**
  Stay lying on the back, hug the right knee and bring across the body to the left side using the left hand. Place right arm out to the side and look towards the right side. Hold for 5-10 breaths and then swap sides.

- **Legs against the wall**
  Lying on the back, come to a wall and lift both legs the wall. Keep the feet around hip-width apart or longer. Place your hands on your belly, close your eyes and let the legs relax, and focus on deep breathing. Stay as long as you want!

Feel there is too much going on

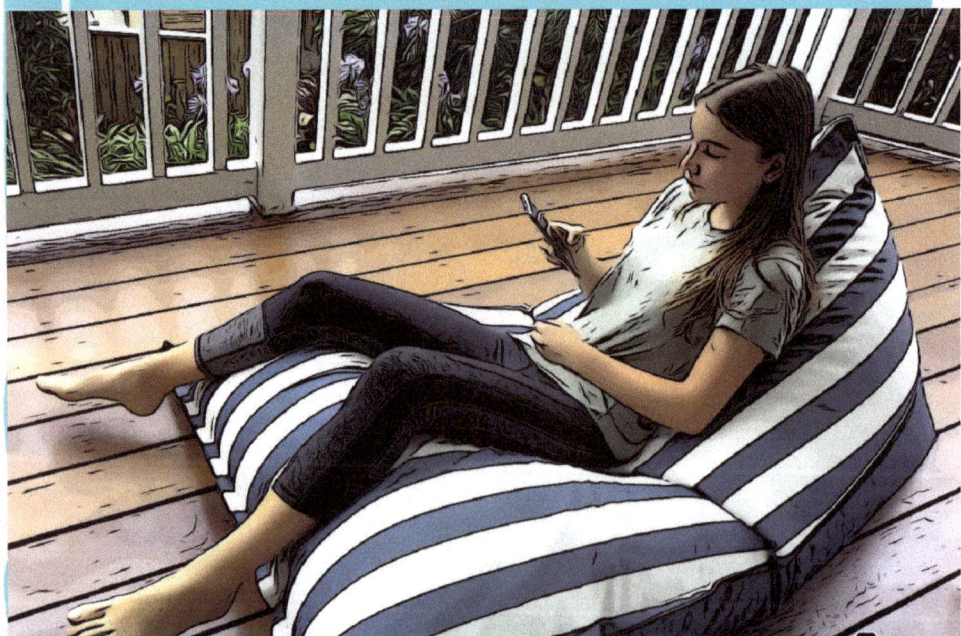

EVER FEEL LIKE THERE IS TOO MUCH GOING ON IN YOUR LIFE?

- Set our own boundaries, and learn to take care of yourself.
- By doing this, it will help with stress levels, our wellbeing, and our relationships.
- If we have too much on, or say YES to everything, we can feel grumpy, super-tired, and get burn-out.
- We can have a more balanced life and do better in school when you learn to say "NO".
- With a more balanced life, it can help lower our stress and anxiety; improve our motivation and energy levels; and boost our confidence and self-esteem.

Make a list if all the things you have happening during the week and the weekends.

Is there anything you could say NO to and create some more balance in your life?

- A great way to have self-care is to start the morning well.

- Eat a healthy breakfast, do even 1-2 minutes of exercise to jump-start your body, do a 5-minute meditation, or add some positive affirmations.

- Throughout the day, carry a water bottle with you to ensure you drink a minimum of 8 glasses of water a day. This will keep you energized through-out the day and also help with memory and con-centration.

- If you have a busy week ahead, plan on a Sunday the week ahead for healthy lunches and dinners. Work with Mum and Dad and ask if you can help do the shopping or cooking for the week.

- When you are making your lunch boxes, take some fruit and vegetables each day and try to keep packaged foods to a minimum.

50-1 BREATH COUNTING

- Great exercise to try to get you to sleep.
- It is also good to use in the middle of the night if you wake up.
- It helps you let go of stress and anxiety, and slows your thoughts down.
- Pick a number – I usually use 50 and then count backward. 50 to 1 will take you around 5 minutes as you are counting each number with the exhale breath. 10 slow breaths usually take around 1 minute.
- If you wake in the middle of the night, maybe even start from 500. Hopefully, you will be definitely asleep by the time you get to 1!

SCARED OR FEARFUL?

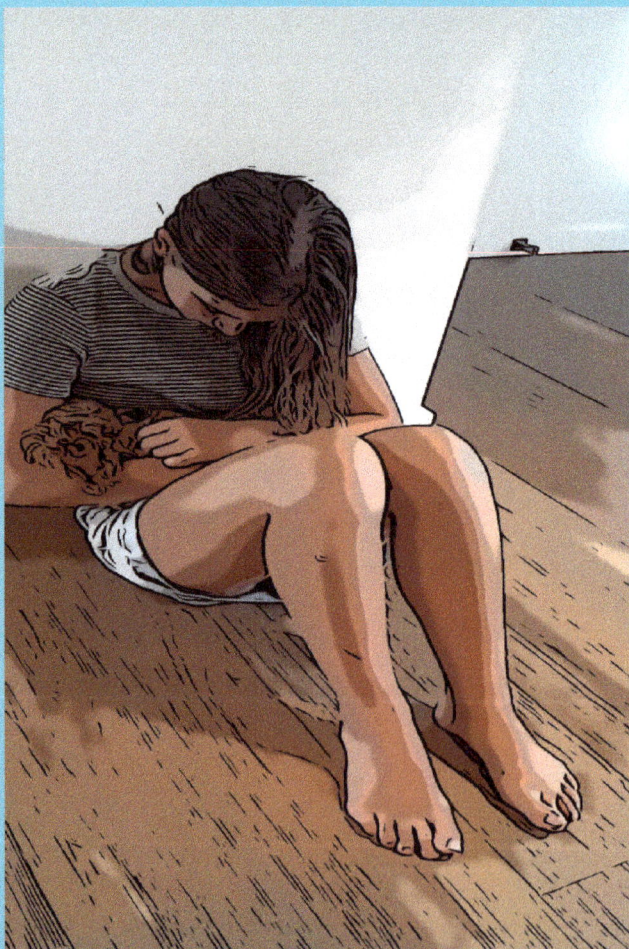

WHAT IS IT LIKE TO HAVE FEAR?

- Unpleasant emotion

- Feeling threat of danger, pain, or harm

- Threat can be real or imagined

- Worst-case scenarios

- Causes physiological and behaviour changes

- Can be important in keeping us safe when in danger

- Becomes a problem when worry takes over the life

- Feeling afraid on a daily basis

- Can be paralysing

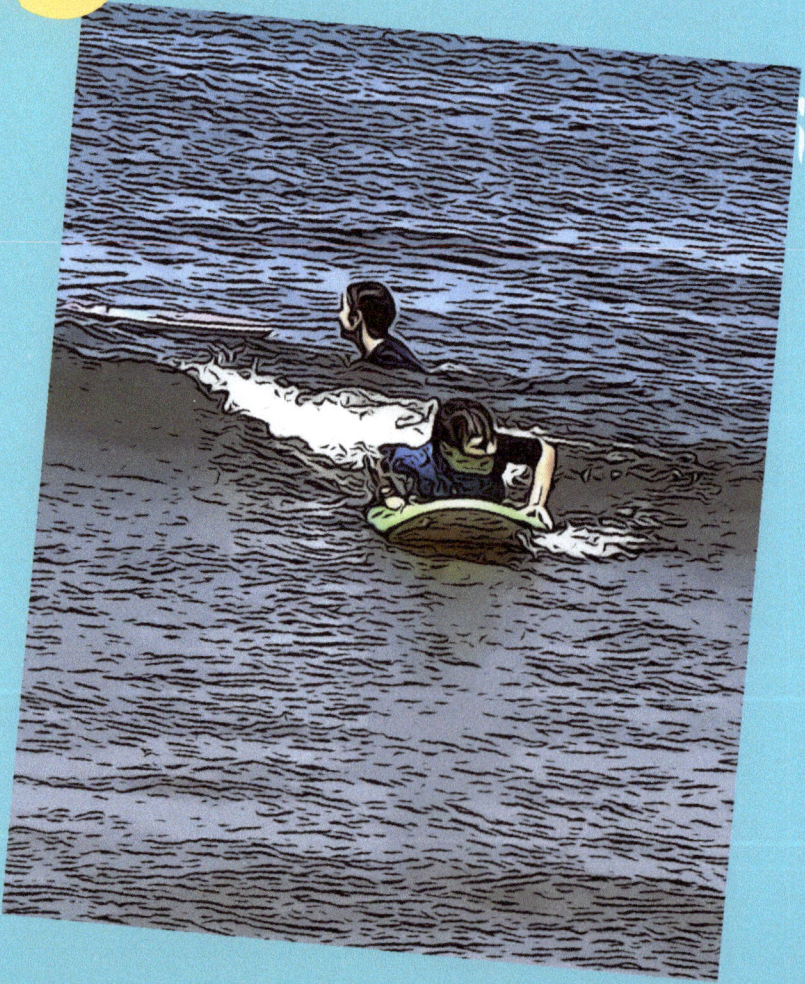

TIPS FOR WHEN YOU FEEL FEAR

- Think of your victories – reverse bucket list of all achieved

- Use breathing techniques for calming

- Come into the here and now - most worries come from the unknown in the future

- Realise your fear – get to the heart of it

- Visualisation best-case scenario

- Fearful thoughts attract more fear – Swap fearful thoughts with positive ones

- Build a support network – friends and family who will listen

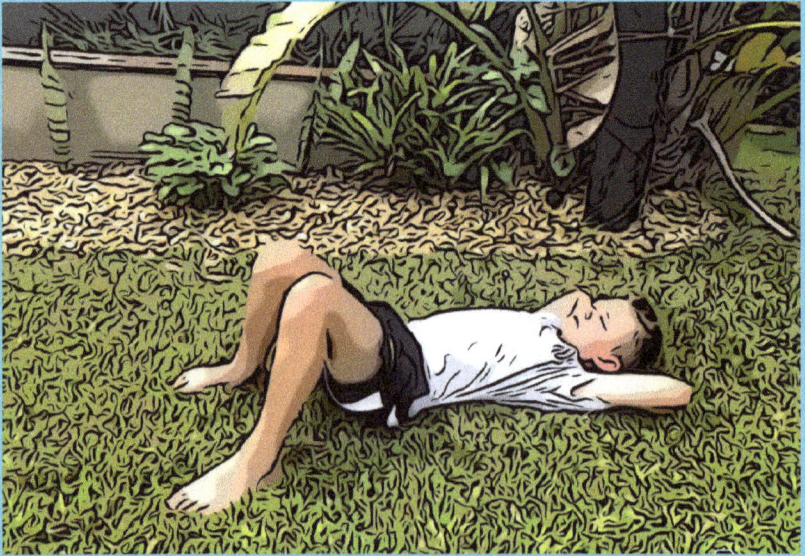

VISUALISE AND USE YOUR IMAGINATION

This can be fun!

- Make a movie about yourself where everything goes perfect.

- Visualise the best-case scenario and the best outcome.

- For example, if you are feeling fear about having to do public speaking in English class, close your eyes, watch yourself walk to the front of the room totally confident and in control. Watch yourself expressing and calming presenting your talk. Notice how you feel as if it is actually happening. Tell yourself you can do this.

- Play this movie in your head and mind as often as you need to before the event you are nervous or worried about.

THINKING OF PAST, WORRIED ABOUT FUTURE?

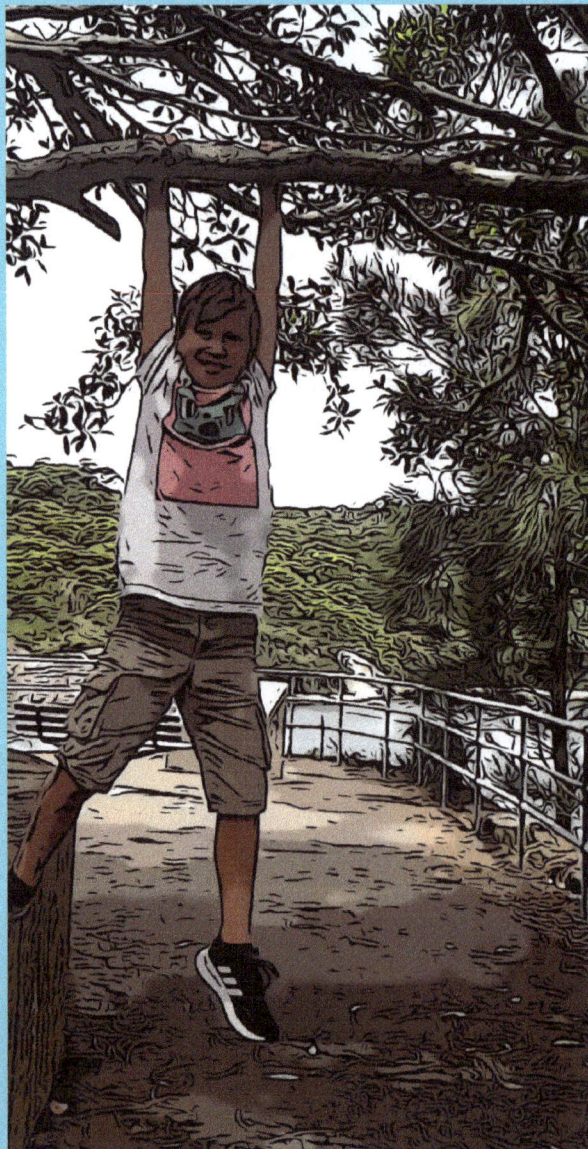

- Want to be in the present, not always thinking of the past, or worries about the future?

- Practicing mindfulness can help you let go of living in the past or future, and bring you to being in the here and now.

- Mindfulness is simply noticing or observing your body, emotions, feelings, thoughts without any judgement on yourself.

- It allows you to focus your awareness on the present moment.

- Be fully present and in the 'here and now, not in the future or past.

- Learn to not over-react or be overwhelmed by what is around us.

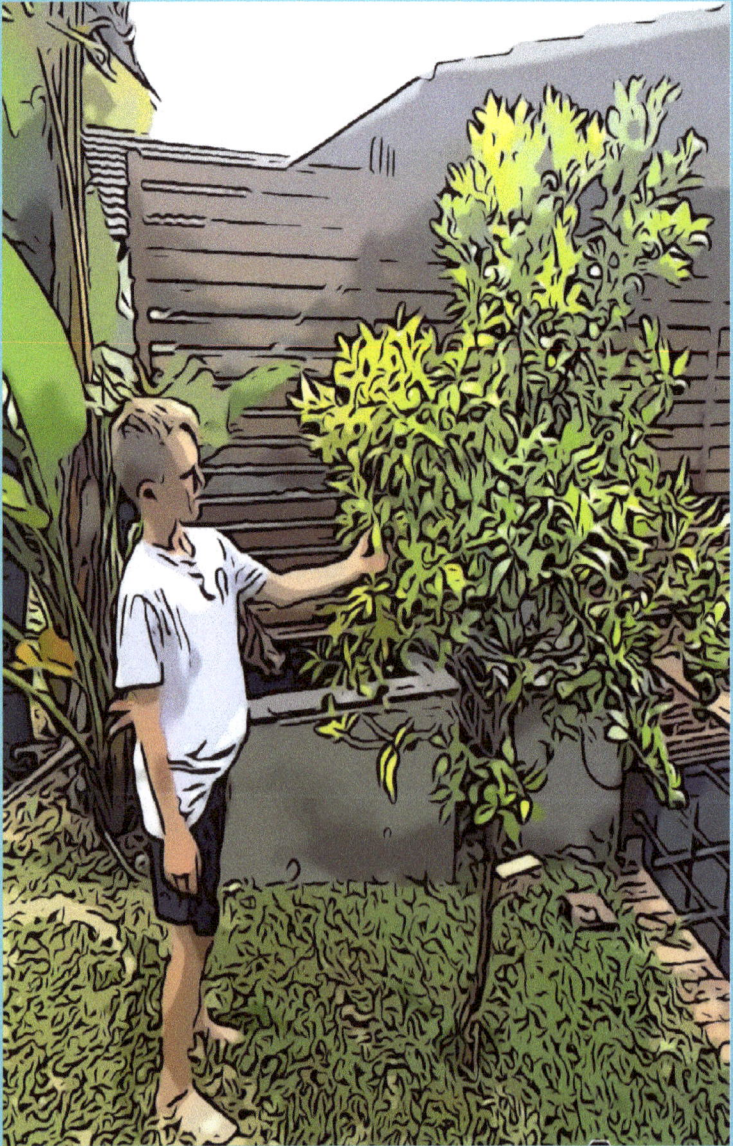

TIPS FOR BEING MINDFUL, NOT HAVING A MIND THAT IS FULL!

- Quiet time each day

- Connect with people

- Enjoy time in nature

- Change up your routine

- Have awe and wonder – notice things around you that are pretty cool! Check out clouds, waves, rainbows, leaves, insects and the list goes on.

- Notice your body and thoughts

- Be grateful each day

- Have a digital detox – even if only half a day!

- Breathe and smile!

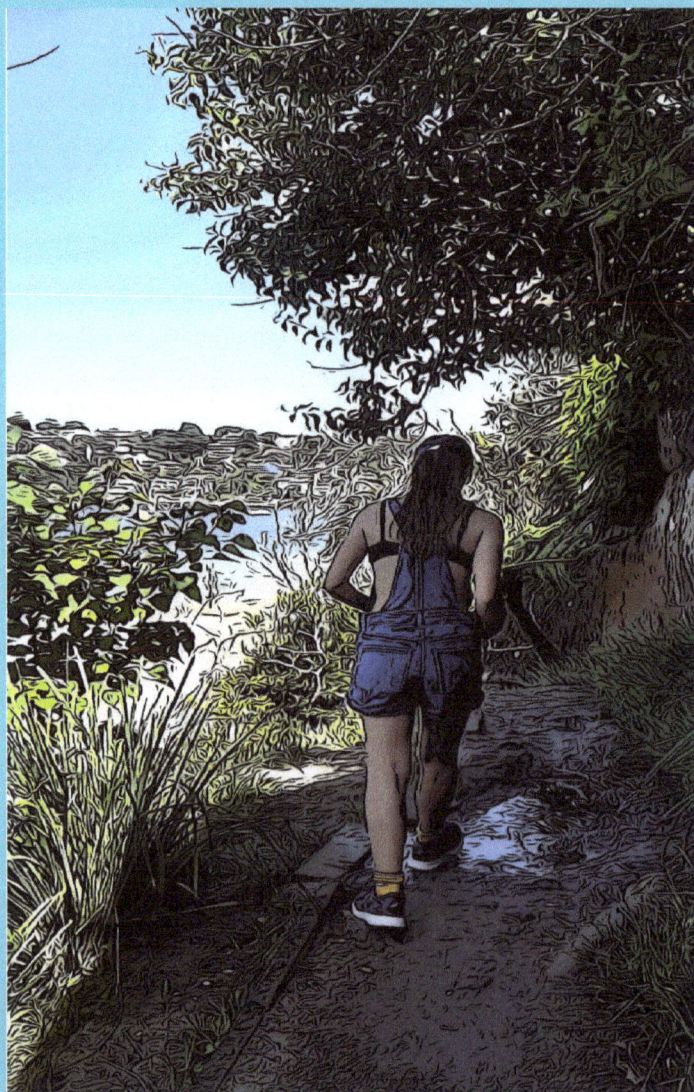

WALKING MEDITATION

- Have a walk without your phone

- Take it slow and notice everything around you

- Use your sense with your surroundings

- For example, how the sand feels underneath your feet on the beach

- OR smelling the leaves in the bush

- OR hearing the kookaburras laughing

- OR feel the sun on your arms

- OR see the birds in the trees above you

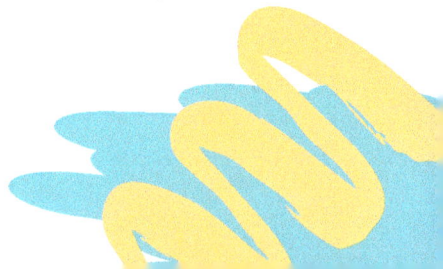

WANT TO FEEL HAPPY AND CALM?

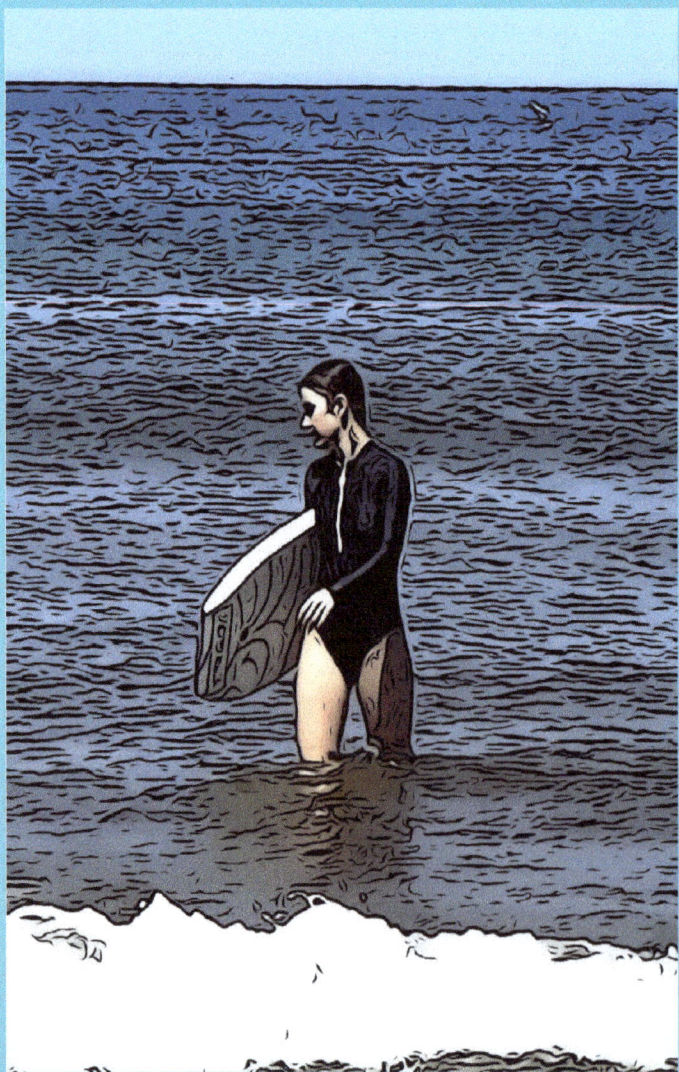

WANT TO FEEL MORE HAPPY AND CALM? TIME TO FIND YOUR FLOW.

The flow state is when we let go of saying in our head - "what's next"?

It is also known as being In the present OR In the now OR In the zone.

Then put the last sentence – Sometimes it is also known as being In the Zone.

Examples of being in the flow are such things as practicing yoga, bushwalking, drawing or painting, walking in nature, hanging out with your pet, surfing, bike riding, baking or cooking, playing or listening to music, or just have a good laugh with your bestie.

When we are in the flow time passes quickly and we feel like we could do that activity every day.

We are being our "true self" rather than someone we think we should be. We are not trying to act cool or a certain way.

MAKE A LIST OF WHAT GETS YOU IN THE FLOW

This list is good to have so that when you are feeling upset, worried or bored, you can try one of these activities.

To get you started, think about the times you have:

- You haven't looked at the time
- You are so caught up in the moment
- You felt great and full of happiness
- You could do this everyday and not get bored
- You are not thinking about what is happening later, or what happened in the past

FIVE SENSES MEDITATION

This is a super easy meditation that you can do anywhere, anytime.

- LOOK: Notice five things you can see
- LISTEN: Notice four sounds you can hear
- FEEL: Notice three distinct sensations
- SMELL: Notice two smells
- TASTE: Notice something you can taste

WANT TO BELIEVE IN YOURSELF?

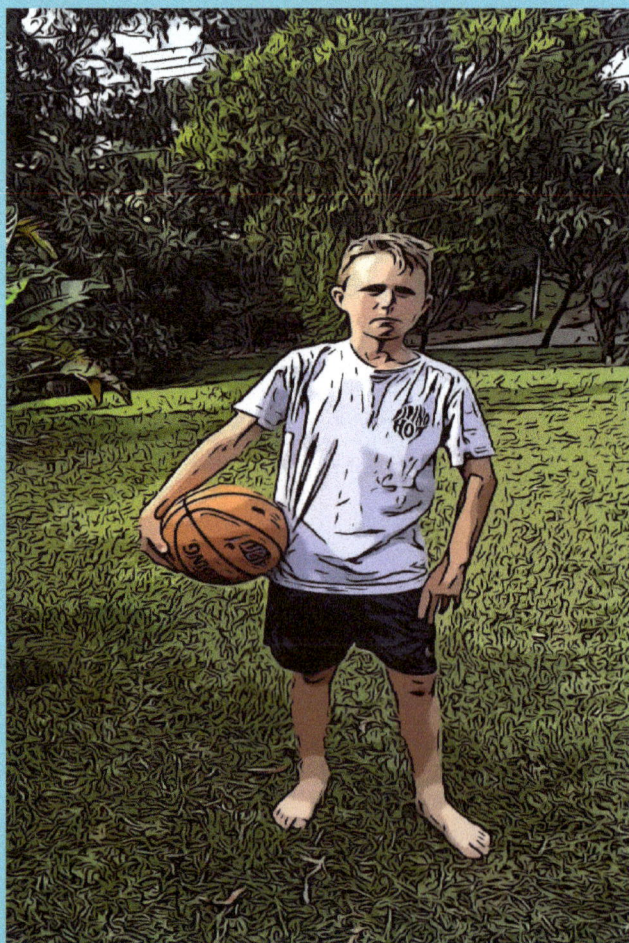

WANT TO BELIEVE IN YOURSELF AND KNOW THAT "YOU CAN DO IT!"

We can change our self-talk using affirmations.

Affirmations are words that affirm what we believe about ourselves. What we think in our minds, creates our reality. Positive thoughts attract positive outcomes, and negative thoughts attract negative outcomes.

For example, imagine you woke up, looked outside and it is raining and cold, and you remembered you had a maths test that day. If you tell yourself (your affirmation) that you are going to have a bad day, you are stressed, and you will do badly in the test, you are increasing the chances of a bad day.

Flip it to say, today is a good day, you are calm, and you will do well in the maths test, what do you think will happen? You have increased your chances of having an awesome day!

WRITE YOUR OWN AFFIRMATIONS

- Think about what is important to you
- What you want to achieve
- How you want to feel
- What are your deepest desires
- How you want to relate to the world
- What about your relationships with friends and family
- How you want to do in school, sport, other activities

Make them:

- Positive
- Personal (I/me)
- Present (as if happening now)
- Passion (put emotion in it)

USE YOUR AFFIRMATIONS

Put them where you can see them. Put them on notes and put them all around the house – like on the fridge, the mirrors in the bathroom, by your bed. Add to breathing 20-40 times a day.

Say each one slowly with each time you breath out. Say them as many times as you can. Like when you first wake up, or on the bus to school, or while you are lying in bed, or cleaning your teeth.

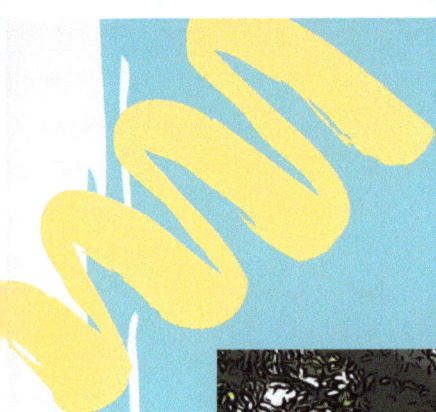

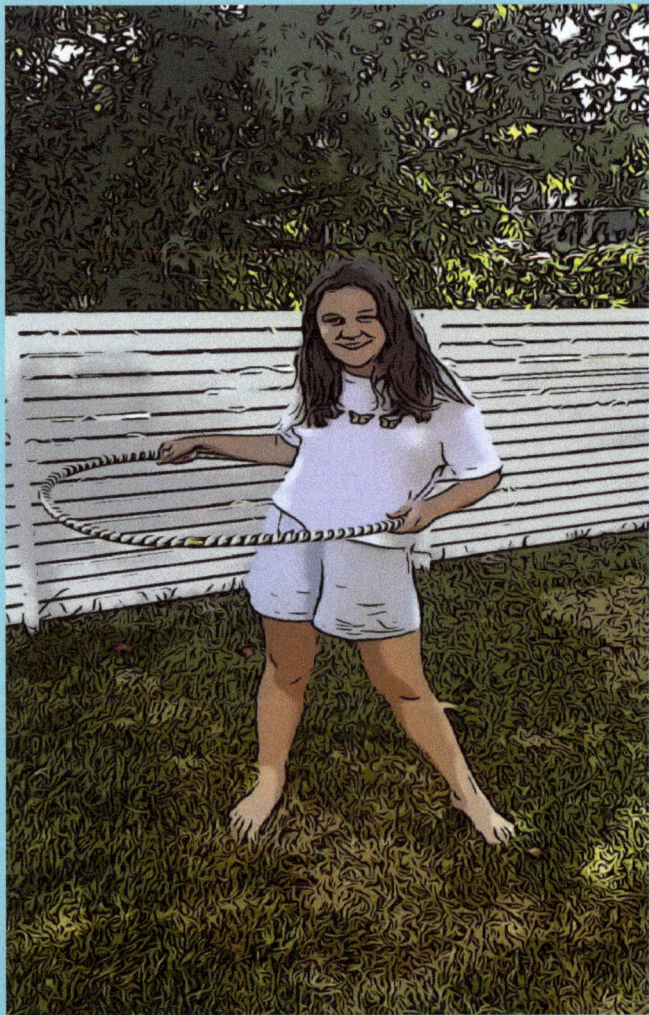

EXAMPLES OF AFFIRMATIONS

- I am smart and clever and am willing to learn when needed
- I am safe and loved
- I am important and my presence is important to myself and others
- I belong and I am loved for exactly who I am
- I believe in myself
- My body is strong and healthy
- I am beautiful and perfect the way I am
- Today is going to be a great day
- I can do this (swim carnival, maths test...)
- I am a good friend
- I am smart and open to learning
- I can make mistakes and still reach my goals

DON'T YOU LOVE YOURSELF AT THE MOMENT?

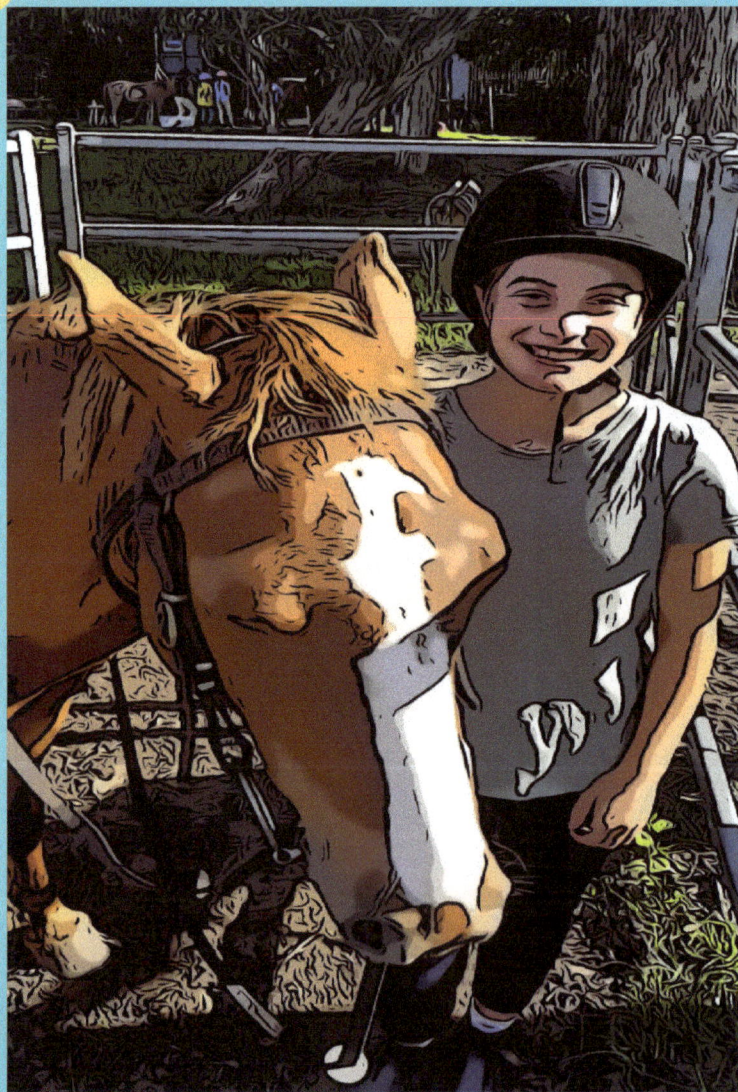

WHY SELF-LOVE IS IMPORTANT

- When you love yourself you can easily give and receive love from others
- Gives you confidence
- Allows you to be resilient in face of adversity
- Helps with failures and overcoming mistakes
- Feel more energised and social – drawn to others
- Feel secure in yourself - helps with relationships
- Helps to let go of feeling worried or anxious

It's good to have self-love! It makes you:

- Proud of who you are
- Have self-esteem and confidence in our worth
- Feel positive about yourself
- Accept compliments
- Be connected to your true self
- Regard for own happiness
- Appreciate and be proud of yourself
- Allows you to follow your own interests and goals

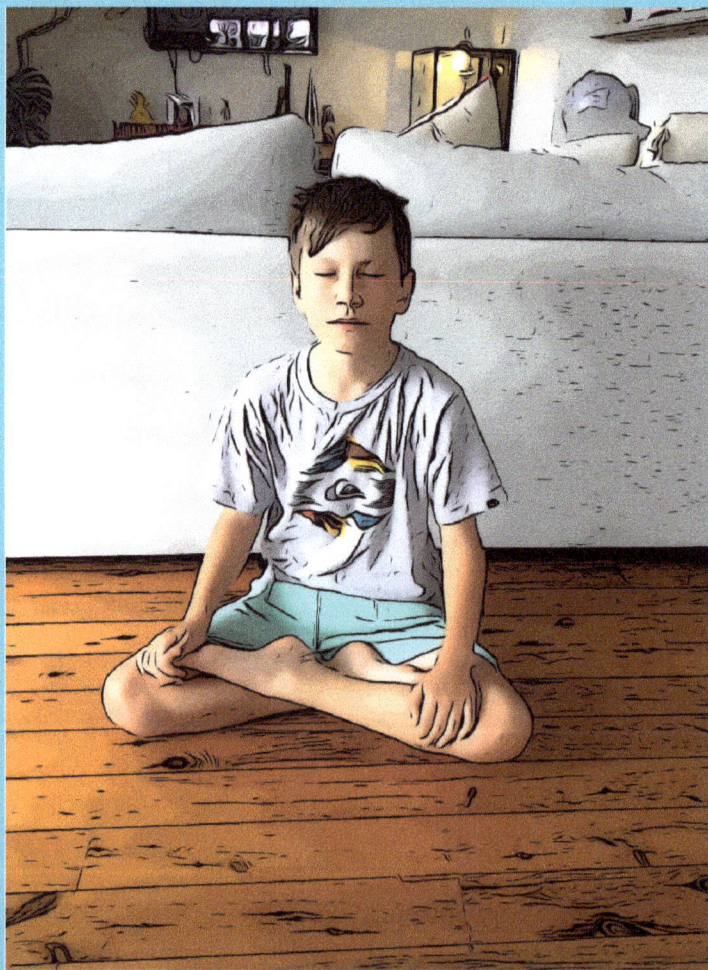

LOVING KINDNESS MEDITATION

Lie down or sit up with your back straight. Close your eyes and take some slow deep breaths.

Say these words in your mind as you picture different people.

I LOVE……, MAY THEY BE SAFE, AND MAY THEY BE HAPPY.

Firstly do this thinking about your family.
Now think about your friends.

Continue with different people in your life – your teachers, neighbours, people you have met in the community.

Next, do this thinking about someone who has hurt you in the past. Even though they have made you upset previously, you still want them to be happy.

Next do this thinking about people all around the world, especially those living in poverty or in a war-zone.

Lastly, picture yourself and send yourself love and say.

I LOVE MYSELF, MAY I BE SAFE, AND MAY I BE HAPPY

FEEL LIKE THERE IS NOTHING GOOD IN YOUR LIFE?

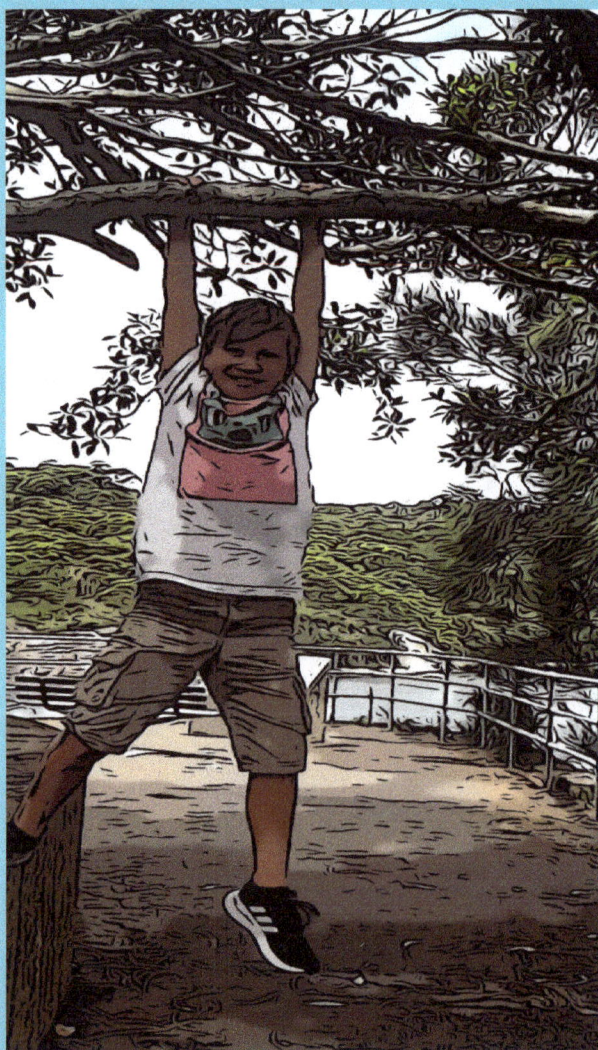

FEEL LIKE THERE'S NOTHING GOOD IN YOUR LIFE? ADDING IN GRATITUDE CAN HELP!

- The word Gratitude comes from the Latin word 'gratis' = pleasing or thankful
- Quality of being thankful
- It is a positive emotion
- It allows you to feel happier
- Make it a daily practice and notice the difference!
- It is an appreciation of all the good in your life
- Gratefulness is a mood, that is also part of your personality
- Can make it a practice – conscious effort
- Leads to a stronger sense of wellbeing

HAVE A HEALTHY MORNING ROUTINE

- Start each morning with some positive affirmations to set you up for a happy day ahead.

- Add some deep breaths, and if you have time, get into nature.

- Be grateful for the simple things – hearing the birds, having your favourite cereal, sport after school.

- See if you can be grateful each morning for three things before you even get out of bed.

GRATITUDE MEDITATION

Notice and appreciate all areas of your life with this meditation. The more you do this, the easier it to realise all the good in your life.

Lie down or sit up with your back straight. Close your eyes and focus on your breath.

We are going to bring attention to different things in our life we can be grateful for.

Firstly, lets are grateful for our senses. What we can hear, smell, taste, see, feel and touch.

Secondly, let's be grateful for the amazing people in your life. Your family, friends, teachers, mentors, coaches, neighbours and anyone that has made your life better by having met them.

Next, let's be grateful for our homes, our possessions, our schools, our hobbies and sports we play, our holidays and our pets.

Lastly, lets are grateful for this moment. Being happy and healthy and alive right now.

Take a deep breath and smile and feel thankful to you for the rest of the day.

CAN'T SWITCH OFF FROM SCREENS?

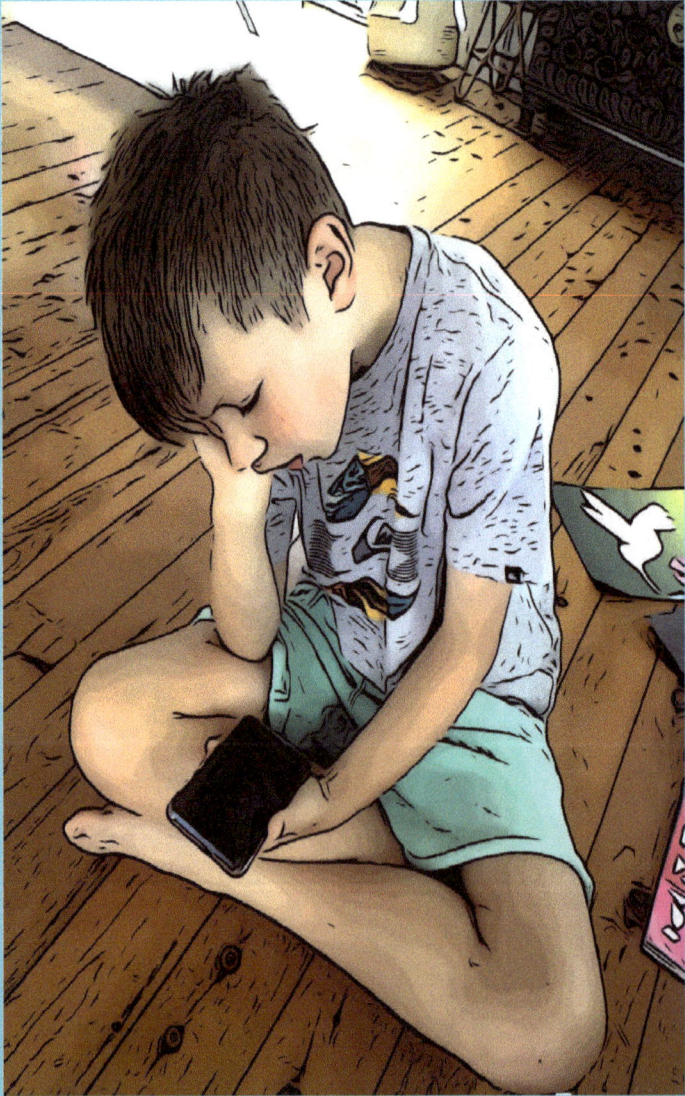

TIPS FOR HAVING A BREAK
FROM OUR DEVICES

- Digital devices are here to complement our lives, not for us to rely on them.

- Try to go for a walk or hang out with friends without a phone.

- Looking at phones before bed interrupts our sleep. Put phone, laptop, and other devices out of the bedroom while you sleep.

- Have a scheduled time in the evening to dis-connect from devices. You can do this by setting an alarm to go off each night, and have some device free time before going to sleep.

- Try to have a digital detox day for half or a full day each week. Plan a fun activity to do with your friends or family instead.

WANT TO FOLLOW YOUR DREAMS?

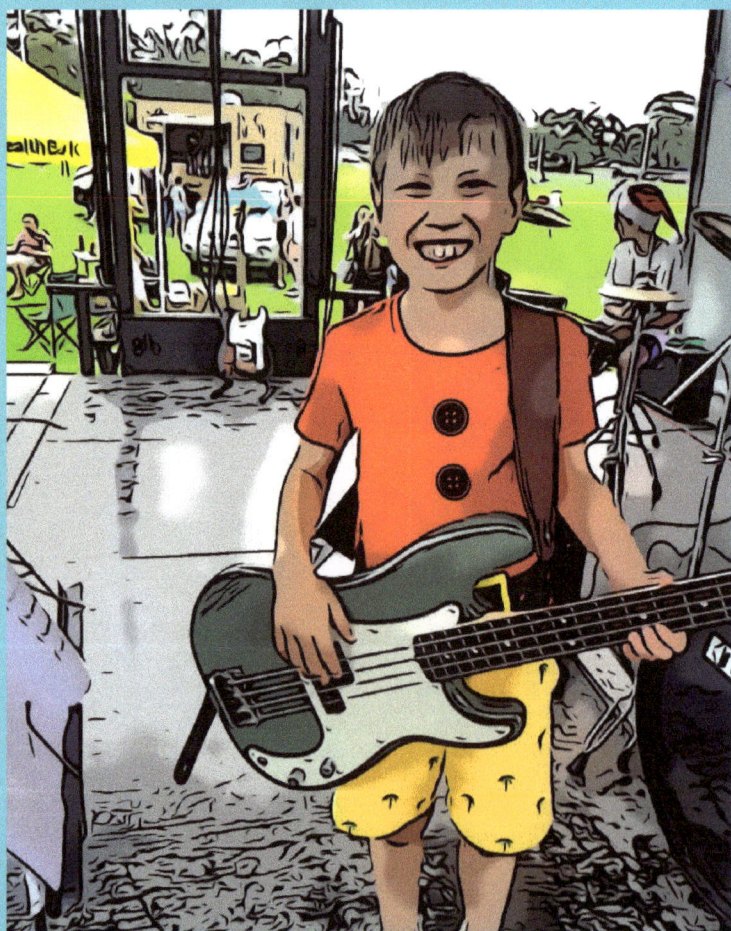

FOLLOW YOUR DREAMS

Many of us are afraid or make excuses as we don't think it is possible to follow our dreams of what we really want to do.

Sometimes you might hear yourself saying things like:

- I'm not good enough
- I don't have enough time
- I'm too young
- I don't have the knowledge or experience
- I've missed the boat here
- I'm too busy
- I don't have what it takes
- I can't afford it
- Clear the excuses and replace negative with positive

ASK, BELIEVE AND RECEIVE

Get a pen and paper and go wild!

Draw, write, cut out pictures out of newspaper or magazine of all your dreams and all the things you want to do in your life!

Now pick one of those dreams and make it into an affirmation (page 72). Write it down as if actually happening to you right now. Imagine how you would feel.

For example, I am a good runner and can run 5km.

Say it like you believe it.

Say it 10 times a day or more. Shout it if you want.

VISUALISATIONS

TRY THIS

Lie down or sit up with your back straight.

Close your eyes and focus on some deep belly breathing.

Now use your imagination. Visualise the best case scenario possible. Imagine you are the star of your own movie where every thing turns out amazing and perfect.

Notice how this feels and do this as much as you need to!
Say your affirmation in your head while you are watching your amazing movie.

FOR EXAMPLE: You are doing a 5km fun run in your visualisation. You are finding it easy, having fun running, and finish the run in a good time. You have a big smile on your face. Also notice what you can see, what you can smell, what you can hear, what you can feel - as if you are actually there right now.

21 DAY CHALLENGE

ARE YOU UP FOR THE CHALLENGE?

It takes a minimum of 21 days to for a habit (some say 66 days, but lets start with 21!)

We are creating a daily check-in habit for our mental health. Even if only for 5 minutes, lets do something that is good for our minds each day.

You have been told to exercise and keep you body healthy, eat fruit and vegetables, clean your teeth each night, put on sunscreen, but it is as equally as important to switch off and create positive habits for your mind.

Start your 21 day MindFlip challenge today!

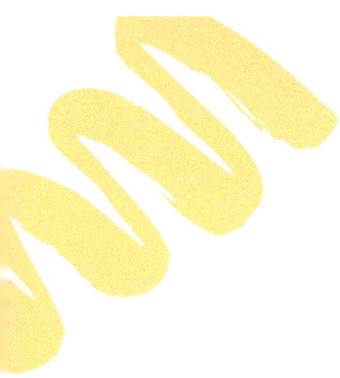

Remember to see how you are talking to yourself and be your own best friend, not your worst enemy!

Small changes to make a big difference

Introduce simple yoga, meditation and breathing exercises.

It is always more fun to do a challenge with a friend. Invite a friend and do it together!

Check out the next pages for breathing, tips, meditation and yoga you can try each day.

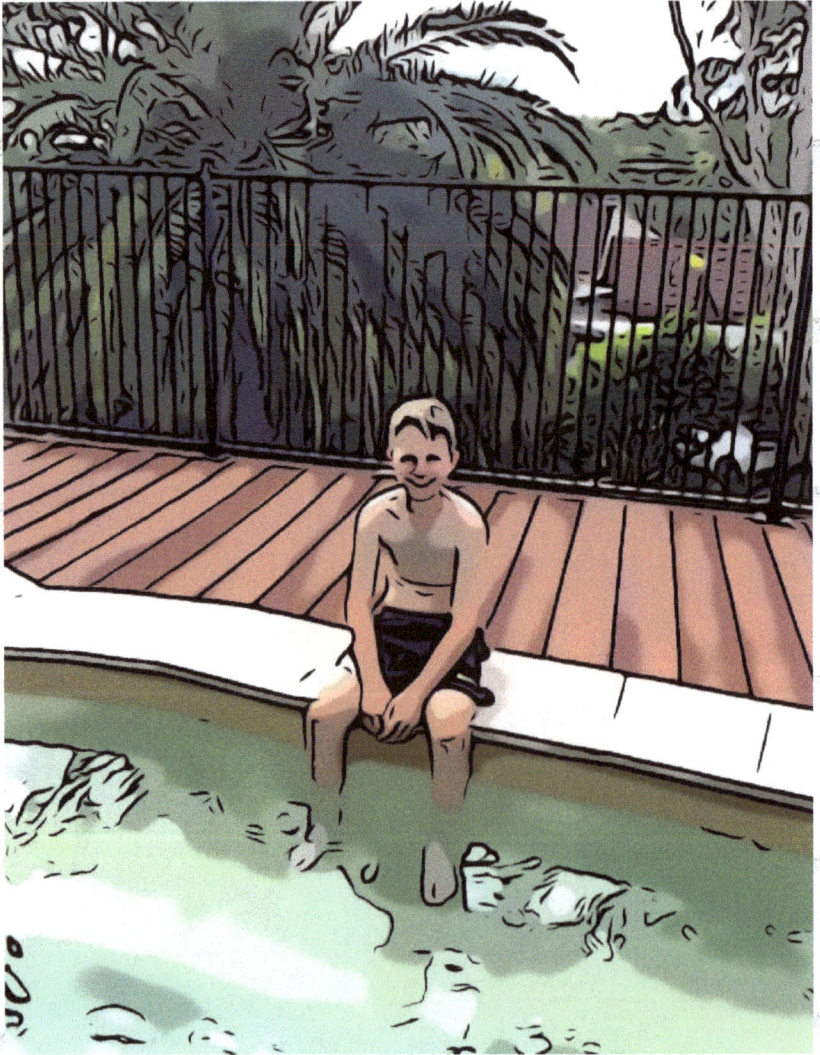

- Write things down

- Recognise stress factors in life and list them

- What are you grateful for

- Set up social support – friends or family

- Take time to laugh

- Regular exercise

- Try yoga or meditation

- Going outdoors

- Forgiving others

- Deep breathing

- Using affirmations and intentions

- Conscious relaxation

BELLY BREATHING

This will help you calm down your mind and make you feel relaxed. Lie down or sit up with back straight, close the eyes and focus on your breathing.

Keep the mouth closed and breath in and out of the nose. Put one hand on your chest and one hand on your belly (under your bellybutton).

Count slowly in your head to four as you breathe in, and then to four as you breathe out. After a few times of this, make the exhale (the out breath) to a count of six, and then if you can to eight if it does not feel uncomfortable.

Keep doing this for a couple of minutes, then let go of the counting and just keep going with the slow breathing.

LEARN TO MEDITATE

Often people think they cannot meditate, or they are doing it wrong as they are unable to stop thinking. Don't worry!

It is not about switching off your thoughts, but about noticing the thoughts and slowing them down.

Try this for a few minutes. Get comfortable and close your eyes. Take a moment to notice your breath going in and out of your nostrils. Tip – keep the mouth closed if you can. After a little while, start to count on the inhale (as you breath in) up to the number 4.

Then on the exhale (as you breath out) see if you can count up the number 6 or even 8. Try this for a few minutes and guess what...you are meditating. Well done!

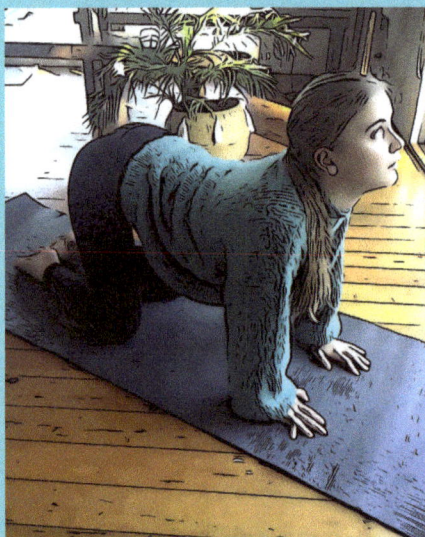
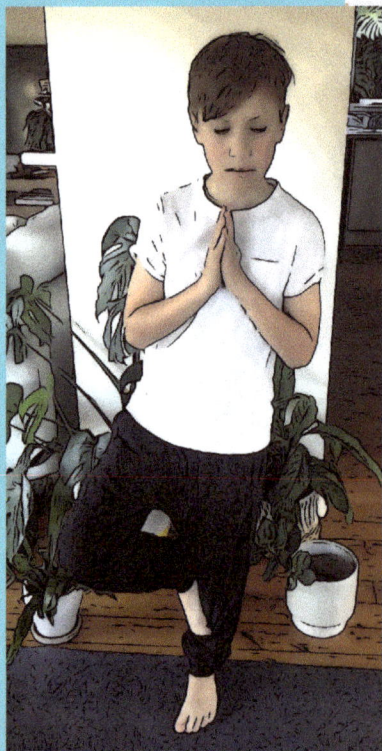
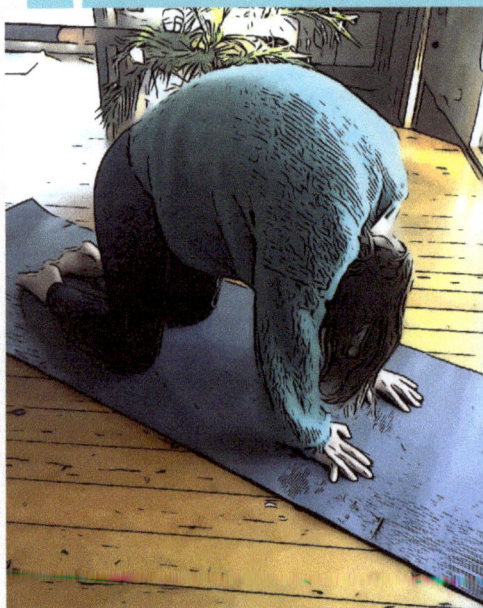
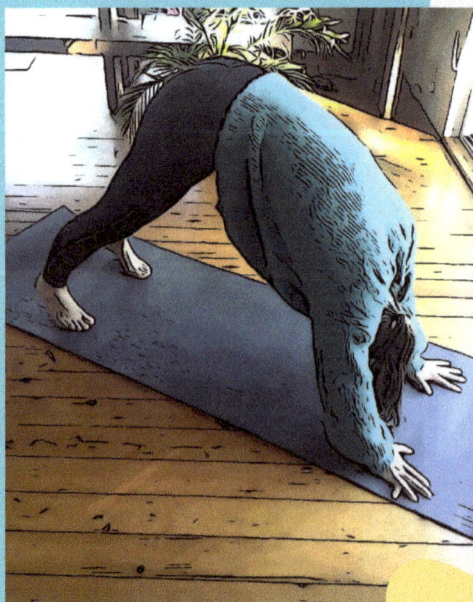

DAILY YOGA POSES

Cat and Cow

Come onto your hands and knees and make a table. Roll the belly down and then look up and breath in slowly. Now roll the other way with the belly up and look towards bellybutton and breath out slowly. Try this 5-10 times

Downward Dog

From table position, lift your hips all the way up to the sky. Look towards the tops of the legs and then try to pull your feet and heels flat on the ground (it does not matter if they do not touch). Your body should look like an upside down V shape. This is an awesome pose for stretching the whole body, giving you energy, your posture and strengthening your arms, legs and core.

Tree pose

Balance on the right foot and place the left foot on the right ankle, calf or up higher above the knee. Bring your arms out to the side for balance or place your hands in prayer pose at your chest. Keep your back straight and look at something that is not moving. Try to hold for 5-10 slow breaths, or longer if you can. Then swap to balancing on the left foot.

Hi, I'm Heidi

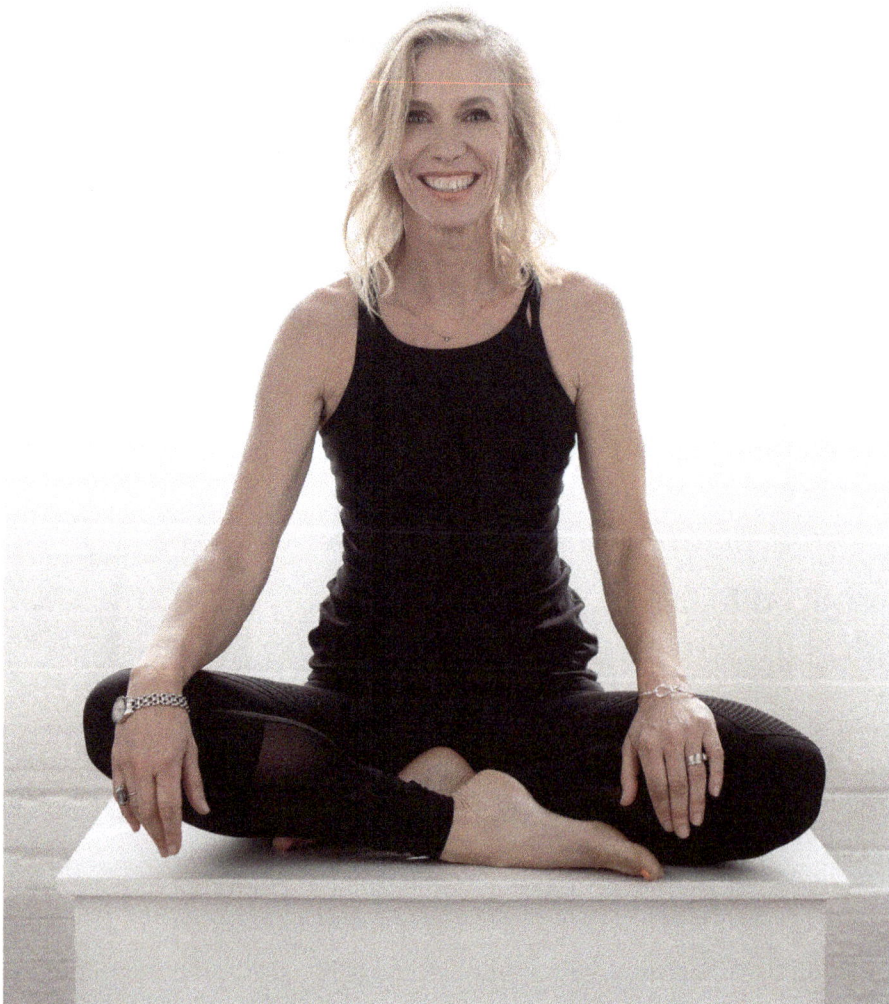

Heidi Horne

Dip Yoga Teacher (Senior Level 3), Wellness Coaching, Life Coaching, Dip Remedial Therapies Counselling and Mental Health (Western Sydney University)

Heidi's yoga and meditation journey began over 25 years ago, and she has been hooked ever since. She loved the feeling yoga created in her physical body, how it calmed her monkey brain (jumping from one thought to another) and how at the end of each session she would feel on top of the world.

As a mum to two children (a tween and a teen), Heidi understands the importance of balance in our busy lives, and how to create a strong and healthy body, as well as a calm and positive mind. As a wellness and mindset specialist, she seeks to guide people through her proven techniques to feel happier, healthier and more positive every day. Heidi is passionate about coaching children to corporates, and shares her expertise of yoga, wellness and mindset to reduce stress and anxiety, and make the everyday extraordinary and fun.

Join Heidi for an ever-evolving journey of self-learning and improvement through mindset, meditation, manifesting, yoga, healthy-living yoga and healthy living. Live a life of purpose and possibilities through her positive mindset coaching programs, key-note speaking, yoga and wellness retreats, corporate/school events, and yoga teacher training.

www.ingramcontent.com/pod-product-compliance
Lightning Source LLC
Chambersburg PA
CBHW041259040426
42334CB00028BA/3090